MONTESSORI FOR DEMENTIA AND OTHER CONDITIONS

BY VERONICA RICCI

ISBN: 9798851585487

Printed in the United States of America

INTRODUCTION TO MONTESSORI APPROACH

A. ORIGINS AND PRINCIPLES OF MONTESSORI EDUCATION

B. ADAPTATION OF MONTESSORI PRINCIPLES FOR DEMENTIA AND OTHER CONDITIONS

The Montessori approach to education, developed by Dr. Maria Montessori in the early 20th century, revolutionized the way we view learning and the potential of every individual. While originally designed for children, the principles and methods of Montessori education have been adapted and found success in various other contexts, including dementia care and other conditions.

Dr. Maria Montessori, an Italian physician and educator, laid the foundation for the Montessori approach in the early 1900s. She observed that children possess an innate drive for learning and emphasized the importance of providing an environment that nurtures their natural curiosity and independence. Dr. Montessori believed that children learn best when given the freedom to explore and engage with their surroundings. This led to the development of the principles that define Montessori education.

At the core of the Montessori approach are the principles of respect for the individual, independence, and self-directed learning. The Montessori classroom is carefully prepared to foster independence and exploration. It features child-sized furniture and materials that are accessible and designed to stimulate the senses and cognitive development. Children are encouraged to choose activities that interest them, engage in uninterrupted work periods, and learn at their own pace. The role of the teacher is that of a facilitator, guiding and supporting the child's learning journey.

The adaptation of Montessori principles for dementia and other conditions is a testament to the flexibility and effectiveness of this approach. Individuals with dementia often experience cognitive decline and challenges with daily tasks. By incorporating Montessori principles into their care, it becomes possible to provide an environment that promotes independence, engagement, and a sense of purpose.

One key aspect of the Montessori approach that is particularly relevant to dementia care is the concept of creating a prepared environment. This involves organizing the physical space in a way that is clear, uncluttered, and familiar to the individual. By incorporating meaningful objects and reducing distractions, the environment can support cognitive functioning and reduce anxiety.

Another essential adaptation is the emphasis on individualized learning and activities. In the Montessori approach, each child's unique needs and interests are taken into account. Similarly, in dementia care, activities and experiences are tailored to the individual's cognitive abilities, preferences, and past interests. This individualized approach ensures that individuals with dementia can engage in activities that are enjoyable, meaningful, and within their capabilities.

The Montessori approach also highlights the importance of sustaining engagement and meaningful social interaction. In dementia care, this translates into creating opportunities for individuals to connect with others, engage in group activities, and foster social connections. Additionally, the approach recognizes the importance of sensory stimulation and cognitive engagement. Activities that incorporate tactile, visual, and auditory stimuli can help stimulate the senses and maintain cognitive functioning.

Implementing the Montessori approach in dementia care requires training and education for caregivers, as well as the adaptation of physical environments in care facilities and homes. Collaboration with healthcare professionals and specialists is crucial to ensure the approach is tailored to the specific needs of individuals with dementia or other conditions. Continuous evaluation and adjustment based on individual progress and changing needs are also essential.

The adaptation of Montessori principles for dementia and other conditions has shown promising results. By enhancing the quality of life, improving cognitive functioning, and reducing behavioral symptoms, the Montessori approach has the potential to transform the care and support provided to individuals with dementia and other conditions.

The Montessori approach, with its origins and principles in child education, has been successfully adapted to support individuals with dementia and other conditions. By creating a prepared environment, promoting independence, providing individualized activities, sustaining engagement and social interaction, and emphasizing sensory stimulation and cognitive engagement, the Montessori approach enhances the well-being and quality of life for those facing cognitive challenges. As we continue to explore and refine the adaptation of Montessori principles, it is evident that person-centered care and individualized approaches are crucial for empowering individuals to thrive despite their conditions.

UNDERSTANDING DEMENTIA AND OTHER CONDITIONS

A. OVERVIEW OF DEMENTIA AND ITS IMPACT ON COGNITIVE ABILITIES

B. OTHER CONDITIONS THAT CAN BENEFIT FROM MONTESSORI APPROACH (E.G., AUTISM, ADHD)

Dementia, a progressive neurological condition, poses significant challenges for individuals and their caregivers. It is characterized by a decline in cognitive abilities, including memory, language, problem-solving, and judgment. However, it is not the only condition that affects cognitive functioning and daily life. Other conditions, such as autism and attention deficit hyperactivity disorder (ADHD), also impact individuals' cognitive processes and can benefit from the Montessori approach.

Dementia is a broad term that encompasses various conditions, the most common of which is Alzheimer's disease. Other types include vascular dementia, Lewy body dementia, and frontotemporal dementia. Regardless of the specific type, dementia affects cognitive abilities, leading to memory loss, difficulties with language and communication, impaired reasoning and judgment, and changes in behavior and personality. As the condition progresses, individuals may require assistance with daily activities and experience challenges in maintaining independence.

Memory loss is one of the defining characteristics of dementia. Individuals may struggle to recall recent events, names of people, or familiar places. This can be frustrating and disorienting, impacting their ability to engage in everyday tasks and maintain social connections. Language difficulties also arise, making it challenging to express thoughts and understand others. Problem-solving and judgment skills decline, affecting decision-making abilities. Changes in behavior, such as agitation, restlessness, and aggression, can emerge as a result of the cognitive decline.

While dementia is a condition that specifically affects older adults, there are other conditions that impact cognitive abilities across different age groups. Autism, a neurodevelopmental disorder, is characterized by challenges in social interaction, communication, and repetitive behaviors. Individuals with autism often experience difficulties with language, social cues, and executive functioning skills. Attention deficit hyperactivity disorder (ADHD) is another condition that affects cognitive functioning, particularly attention, impulse control, and hyperactivity. Individuals with ADHD may struggle with focusing on tasks, staying organized, and managing their behavior.

The Montessori approach, originally designed for children, has demonstrated its adaptability and effectiveness in supporting individuals with dementia as well as those with other conditions. The principles and methods of Montessori education can be applied to create supportive environments and tailored activities for individuals with autism, ADHD, and other cognitive conditions.

In the Montessori approach, creating a prepared environment plays a crucial role. This concept involves organizing the physical space in a way that supports independence, exploration, and learning. For individuals with autism, this may involve incorporating sensory elements and providing structured and predictable spaces. For individuals with ADHD, it may involve minimizing distractions and creating clear visual cues to help with focus and organization.

Individualized learning and activities are key components of the Montessori approach. By assessing each individual's unique strengths, interests, and abilities, activities can be tailored to their specific needs and preferences. For individuals with autism, this may involve providing activities that match their sensory preferences and promoting social interactions in a structured and supportive manner. For individuals with ADHD, it may involve breaking tasks into manageable steps and offering hands-on, engaging activities to enhance focus and attention.

Sustaining engagement and meaningful social interaction is another important aspect of the Montessori approach. For individuals with autism, this can involve creating opportunities for structured social interactions and fostering connections with peers. For individuals with ADHD, it may involve incorporating movement and interactive elements into learning activities to maintain engagement and facilitate social connections.

The Montessori approach also emphasizes sensory stimulation and cognitive engagement. This is particularly relevant for individuals with autism, as sensory experiences play a significant role in their perception and understanding of the world. Providing a variety of sensory-rich activities can enhance their cognitive functioning and overall well-being. For individuals with ADHD, incorporating hands-on and interactive learning experiences can stimulate their attention and cognitive engagement.

While dementia is a condition that significantly impacts cognitive abilities and daily life, other conditions such as autism and ADHD also affect individuals' cognitive functioning. The Montessori approach, with its emphasis on creating a prepared environment, individualized learning, sustaining engagement and meaningful social interaction, as well as sensory stimulation and cognitive engagement, has demonstrated its applicability and effectiveness in supporting individuals with various cognitive conditions. By adapting the principles and methods of Montessori education, individuals with autism, ADHD, and other cognitive conditions can benefit from a supportive and empowering approach that enhances their overall well-being and cognitive development.

MONTESSORI PRINCIPLES APPLIED TO DEMENTIA AND OTHER CONDITIONS

A. CREATING A PREPARED ENVIRONMENT

The Montessori approach, originally designed for children, has shown great potential in supporting individuals with dementia and other conditions. One fundamental aspect of the Montessori approach is the creation of a prepared environment that promotes independence, engagement, and a sense of purpose.

Creating clear and organized spaces is essential for individuals with dementia and other conditions. Cluttered and disorganized environments can be overwhelming and confusing, leading to increased anxiety and agitation. By providing a clear and structured physical space, individuals can navigate their surroundings more easily, which can help reduce stress and promote a sense of calm.

In a Montessori-inspired environment, furniture and materials are arranged in a logical and accessible manner. For individuals with dementia, this means ensuring that pathways are clear, furniture is arranged for ease of movement, and objects are within reach. Clear labels and visual cues can also be used to aid navigation and promote independence.

Incorporating familiar and meaningful objects is another crucial aspect of the prepared environment for individuals with dementia and other conditions. Familiar objects can evoke positive memories and provide a sense of comfort and security. By including personal belongings, photographs, and items that hold emotional significance, the environment becomes more personalized and meaningful.

In a Montessori approach to dementia care, objects that have practical use and familiarity, such as kitchen utensils or tools, can be incorporated into activities that promote engagement and cognitive stimulation. For individuals with conditions like autism or ADHD, familiar objects and materials that align with their interests and sensory preferences can be included to facilitate learning and engagement.

Reducing clutter and distractions is vital in supporting individuals with dementia and other conditions. Excessive visual and auditory stimuli can lead to sensory overload and difficulties in focusing. By minimizing unnecessary objects and noise, the environment becomes more conducive to concentration and engagement in meaningful activities.

In a Montessori-inspired environment, clutter is kept to a minimum, and materials are organized and neatly displayed. This allows individuals to focus on one activity at a time and reduces the potential for confusion or distraction. Removing unnecessary items and simplifying the environment also supports individuals with conditions like autism or ADHD, enabling them to process information more effectively and engage in tasks without being overwhelmed.

Moreover, reducing distractions in the environment helps individuals with dementia maintain a sense of continuity and a connection to their present reality. By minimizing visual and auditory distractions, caregivers can create a more supportive environment that allows individuals to concentrate on tasks and interactions.

The Montessori principles of creating a prepared environment have significant applications in supporting individuals with dementia and other conditions. Clear and organized spaces help individuals navigate their surroundings with ease, while incorporating familiar and meaningful objects provides comfort and stimulation. Furthermore, reducing clutter and distractions promotes concentration and engagement. By adapting the Montessori approach to dementia and other conditions, caregivers can provide individuals with environments that support their independence, engagement, and overall well-being.

B. PROMOTING INDEPENDENCE AND AUTONOMY

Promoting independence and autonomy is a fundamental aspect of the Montessori approach, and its significance becomes even more pronounced when applied to individuals with dementia and other conditions. Empowering individuals to maintain their sense of self and agency in their daily lives is crucial for their overall well-being and quality of life.

Dementia and other conditions can significantly impact individuals' cognitive abilities and daily functioning. As these conditions progress, individuals may face challenges in completing routine tasks, making decisions, and maintaining a sense of control over their lives. However, it is essential to recognize and respect their inherent need for independence and autonomy.

The Montessori approach recognizes that independence fosters a sense of purpose, accomplishment, and self-esteem. When individuals are given the opportunity to engage in activities on their terms and at their own pace, they can experience a renewed sense of agency and dignity. This approach aligns well with the philosophy of person-centered care, which aims to prioritize the individual's needs, preferences, and abilities.

In the context of dementia, promoting independence and autonomy involves creating an environment that supports the individual's capabilities and encourages self-care. For example, organizing the physical space in a way that allows individuals to easily access personal items or engage in everyday tasks independently is crucial. This could include labeling drawers, arranging items in an orderly manner, and providing clear instructions or visual cues.

Incorporating familiar objects and routines further enhances independence and autonomy. Individuals with dementia often respond positively to activities or objects that have personal significance. By incorporating familiar items, such as family photographs, treasured possessions, or items related to their past interests or profession, individuals can engage in meaningful activities that boost their confidence and preserve their identity.

The Montessori approach also emphasizes providing choices and opportunities for decision-making. This is particularly relevant for individuals with conditions such as autism or ADHD, as they may struggle with decision-making and maintaining focus. By offering a range of options and respecting individual preferences, caregivers can empower individuals to make meaningful choices and exercise their autonomy.

Engaging in purposeful activities is another key component of promoting independence and autonomy. By incorporating tasks that align with individuals' interests and abilities, they can actively participate in their own care and contribute to their daily routines. These activities can range from self-care tasks, such as dressing or grooming, to engaging in hobbies or crafts that provide a sense of accomplishment.

Promoting independence and autonomy goes beyond physical tasks. It also involves fostering a supportive and respectful environment where individuals feel heard and valued. Caregivers can actively involve individuals in decision-making processes, encourage their input, and respect their choices. This collaborative approach empowers individuals to maintain a sense of control and self-determination.

The benefits of promoting independence and autonomy extend beyond individual well-being. When individuals with dementia and other conditions are given opportunities to engage in meaningful activities and exercise their autonomy, they are more likely to experience a sense of purpose, reduce behavioral symptoms, and maintain cognitive functioning to the best of their abilities. Moreover, caregivers can also benefit from a reduced burden of care as individuals become more self-sufficient and actively contribute to their daily lives.

By creating an environment that supports their capabilities, providing choices and opportunities for decision-making, engaging in purposeful activities, and fostering a respectful and collaborative approach, caregivers can empower individuals to maintain their sense of self and agency. This not only enhances their overall well-being and quality of life but also contributes to a more inclusive and person-centered approach to care.

C. INDIVIDUALIZED LEARNING AND ACTIVITIES

The Montessori approach emphasizes the importance of recognizing and valuing the unique strengths, interests, and abilities of each individual. When applying this approach to individuals with dementia and other conditions, it becomes crucial to assess their cognitive abilities, preferences, and sensory needs.

Assessing individual strengths, interests, and abilities is a fundamental step in providing person-centered care. It involves understanding the unique characteristics and capabilities of each individual, enabling caregivers to design activities that are meaningful, engaging, and aligned with their abilities.

For individuals with dementia, cognitive abilities may vary depending on the stage and type of dementia. It is crucial to conduct a comprehensive assessment to identify their strengths, such as preserved memories, retained skills, and areas of interest. This assessment can involve conversations with the individual, family members, and healthcare professionals, as well as observations of their behavior and engagement in various activities.

By tailoring activities to match cognitive abilities and preferences, caregivers can provide opportunities for individuals to engage in tasks that are within their capabilities and offer a sense of accomplishment. For example, if an individual enjoys gardening, they can participate in simple gardening activities, such as planting seeds or tending to potted plants. If an individual has a background in music, they may enjoy participating in music therapy or engaging in activities that involve listening to or playing musical instruments.

Tailoring activities based on preferences extends beyond their interests. It also involves adapting activities to accommodate their preferred learning style, sensory preferences, and personal routines. For example, some individuals may thrive in a structured and predictable environment, while others may prefer a more flexible and spontaneous approach. By respecting individual preferences, caregivers can create a supportive and comfortable environment that enhances engagement and promotes a sense of well-being.

Offering a variety of multi-sensory experiences is another important aspect of the Montessori approach when working with individuals with dementia and other conditions. Multi-sensory experiences engage individuals through multiple senses, stimulating their cognitive functioning and creating meaningful connections. This can involve incorporating tactile, visual, auditory, and olfactory stimuli into activities.

For individuals with dementia, multi-sensory experiences can help evoke memories, promote cognitive engagement, and enhance well-being. For example, engaging in reminiscence therapy by providing items with distinct textures, scents, or sounds associated with their past can facilitate connections to positive memories. Engaging in art activities that involve touch, such as sculpting or painting, can provide tactile stimulation and promote self-expression.

In the case of other conditions, such as autism or ADHD, multi-sensory experiences can also be beneficial. Individuals with autism often respond well to visual and tactile stimuli, while individuals with ADHD may benefit from activities that engage multiple senses to promote focus and concentration.

By offering a variety of multi-sensory experiences, caregivers can cater to different individuals' preferences and provide a holistic and enriching environment. This variety helps prevent monotony, maintains interest, and supports cognitive development and emotional well-being.

When applying the Montessori approach to individuals with dementia and other conditions, it is crucial to assess their strengths, interests, and abilities. By tailoring activities to match their cognitive abilities and preferences, caregivers can create meaningful and engaging experiences that promote a sense of accomplishment and well-being. Additionally, offering a variety of multi-sensory experiences enhances cognitive stimulation and fosters connections. By embracing individuality and adapting activities accordingly, caregivers can provide a person-centered approach that respects and celebrates the unique qualities of each individual.

D. SUSTAINING ENGAGEMENT AND MEANINGFUL SOCIAL INTERACTION

The Montessori method emphasizes the importance of social connections and interactions in fostering holistic development and well-being. When applying the Montessori approach to individuals with dementia and other conditions, facilitating social connections, incorporating group activities and discussions, and providing opportunities for intergenerational interactions become essential elements.

Facilitating social connections and peer interactions is crucial for individuals with dementia and other conditions, as it enhances their overall well-being and quality of life. Human connection plays a vital role in maintaining cognitive functioning, emotional resilience, and a sense of belonging. By creating opportunities for individuals to engage in social interactions, caregivers can help combat feelings of isolation and loneliness that individuals with dementia and other conditions often experience.

In a Montessori-inspired approach, facilitating social connections involves creating a supportive and inclusive environment where individuals can engage with peers, family members, and caregivers. This can be achieved through various means, such as organizing group activities, promoting collaborative projects, and establishing regular social gatherings. By encouraging individuals to participate in these social interactions, caregivers can help individuals maintain and develop their social skills, foster a sense of community, and reduce the negative impact of isolation.

Incorporating group activities and discussions is another important component when applying the Montessori method to individuals with dementia and other conditions. Group activities provide a platform for individuals to engage with others, share experiences, and learn from one another. These activities can include group exercises, games, art projects, or even group outings.

In a group setting, individuals can benefit from the collective wisdom, support, and shared experiences. For individuals with dementia, group activities and discussions can help stimulate cognitive functioning, encourage socialization, and foster a sense of belonging. Group interactions can also provide opportunities for individuals to practice communication skills, problem-solving, and cooperation.

Providing opportunities for intergenerational interactions adds another layer of enrichment when applying the Montessori method to individuals with dementia and other conditions. Interactions with individuals from different generations offer unique perspectives, valuable connections, and meaningful relationships.

Intergenerational interactions can be facilitated through various means, such as organizing intergenerational activities or fostering connections with local schools or community organizations. For example, individuals with dementia can engage in joint activities with children, such as storytelling, arts and crafts, or gardening. These interactions not only provide cognitive and emotional stimulation but also offer a sense of purpose and fulfillment through sharing knowledge and experiences with younger generations.

Intergenerational interactions also benefit individuals with conditions such as autism or ADHD. The presence of children can create a dynamic and engaging environment that stimulates social interactions, encourages communication, and enhances emotional well-being.

When applying the Montessori method to individuals with dementia and other conditions, facilitating social connections, incorporating group activities and discussions, and providing opportunities for intergenerational interactions are vital aspects. These elements foster engagement, emotional well-being, and a sense of belonging in individuals who may otherwise experience feelings of isolation and loneliness. By creating a supportive and inclusive environment that values social connections, caregivers can enhance the overall quality of life and promote holistic development in individuals with dementia and other conditions. The Montessori method, with its focus on person-centered care and meaningful interactions, provides a framework for creating a sense of community, promoting social engagement, and nurturing relationships across generations.

E. EMPHASIZING SENSORY STIMULATION AND COGNITIVE ENGAGEMENT

The Montessori method recognizes the importance of sensory stimulation and cognitive engagement in promoting overall well-being and development. When applying the Montessori approach to individuals with dementia and other conditions, incorporating tactile, visual, and auditory stimuli, engaging in cognitive exercises and brain-stimulating activities, and modifying activities as the condition progresses become essential elements.

Incorporating tactile, visual, and auditory stimuli is a crucial component of the Montessori method when working with individuals with dementia and other conditions. Sensory experiences play a vital role in stimulating cognitive functioning, evoking memories, and enhancing overall engagement. By providing a multi-sensory environment, caregivers can create meaningful and enriching experiences for individuals.

For individuals with dementia, incorporating tactile stimuli involves providing materials and activities that involve touch and texture. This can include objects with varying textures, such as fabrics, natural materials, or tactile puzzles. By engaging the sense of touch, individuals can maintain sensory stimulation, promote motor skills, and enhance their connection to the world around them.

Visual stimuli are also significant in supporting individuals with dementia and other conditions. Using visual cues and aids, such as clear and visual instructions, visual aids, or visual schedules, can help individuals understand tasks and routines more easily. Incorporating art activities, such as painting or coloring, or displaying visual stimuli, such as artwork or photographs, can provide visual stimulation and evoke emotions and memories.

Auditory stimuli are equally important in engaging individuals and promoting cognitive functioning. Music therapy, for example, has been shown to have a positive impact on individuals with dementia, stimulating memories, improving mood, and facilitating social interactions. Incorporating auditory elements, such as listening to familiar songs, engaging in discussions or storytelling, or providing auditory cues, can enhance cognitive engagement and emotional well-being.

Engaging in cognitive exercises and brain-stimulating activities is another significant aspect of the Montessori method when working with individuals with dementia and other conditions. These exercises promote mental agility, memory recall, problem-solving skills, and overall cognitive functioning. Cognitive exercises can involve puzzles, memory games, word association tasks, or any activity that challenges cognitive abilities.

For individuals with conditions like autism or ADHD, engaging in brain-stimulating activities is equally important. These activities can involve logical thinking puzzles, math problems, or tasks that require attention, concentration, and problem-solving. By engaging in such activities, individuals can develop and strengthen cognitive skills, improve focus, and enhance overall cognitive functioning.

As conditions progress, it becomes essential to modify activities to accommodate changing needs and abilities. The Montessori approach recognizes the individuality of each person and acknowledges that their capabilities may change over time. Caregivers need to adapt activities to ensure they remain challenging and engaging while still being within the individual's capabilities.

Modifications can involve simplifying tasks, providing additional support, breaking activities into smaller steps, or offering alternative options. For example, if an individual with dementia enjoys painting but struggles with fine motor skills, providing larger brushes or using adaptive tools can enable them to continue engaging in artistic activities. For individuals with conditions like autism or ADHD, modifying activities can involve adjusting the level of difficulty or providing additional structure and support to ensure successful participation.

When using the Montessori method for individuals with dementia and other conditions, incorporating tactile, visual, and auditory stimuli, engaging in cognitive exercises and brain-stimulating activities, and modifying activities as the condition progresses are crucial elements. These aspects enhance cognitive functioning, promote emotional well-being, and accommodate changing needs. By creating a multi-sensory environment, engaging in brain-stimulating activities, and adapting activities to individual capabilities, caregivers can provide meaningful and enriching experiences that promote cognitive engagement and overall well-being. The Montessori method's focus on individualized care and continuous adaptation ensures that individuals with dementia and other conditions receive tailored support that respects their unique needs and abilities throughout their journey.

IMPLEMENTING THE MONTESSORI APPROACH

A. TRAINING AND EDUCATION FOR CAREGIVERS

B. ADAPTING PHYSICAL ENVIRONMENTS IN CARE FACILITIES AND HOMES

C. COLLABORATING WITH HEALTHCARE PROFESSIONALS AND SPECIALISTS

D. EVALUATING AND ADJUSTING THE APPROACH BASED ON INDIVIDUAL NEEDS

Implementing the Montessori approach with individuals with dementia and other conditions requires careful planning, training, and collaboration among caregivers, healthcare professionals, and specialists.

Training and education for caregivers is a vital aspect of implementing the Montessori approach effectively. Caregivers need to develop a thorough understanding of the principles, philosophy, and methods of the Montessori approach. This includes knowledge of the specific needs, challenges, and capabilities of individuals with dementia and other conditions.

Caregivers should receive training on how to create a prepared environment, tailor activities to individual needs, promote independence and autonomy, facilitate social connections, and incorporate multi-sensory experiences. They should also be trained in effective communication strategies, problem-solving techniques, and conflict resolution to ensure a supportive and person-centered approach.

In addition to training, ongoing education and professional development opportunities are crucial to keep caregivers updated with the latest research and best practices in the field of dementia and other conditions.

Regular training sessions, workshops, and peer support groups can help caregivers enhance their skills and stay informed about advancements in care approaches.

Adapting physical environments in care facilities and homes is another essential element of implementing the Montessori approach. The physical environment plays a significant role in supporting individuals' independence, engagement, and well-being. Careful attention should be given to the layout, organization, and design of spaces to ensure they are safe, accessible, and conducive to individuals' needs and preferences.

Adapting physical environments involves creating clear pathways, minimizing clutter, and ensuring that materials and objects are easily accessible. Caregivers should consider incorporating familiar and meaningful objects, clear signage and labeling, and visual cues to aid individuals' navigation and promote independence. Adjustments should also be made to accommodate sensory preferences, such as incorporating calming or stimulating elements based on individuals' sensory needs.

Collaboration with healthcare professionals and specialists is crucial for successful implementation of the Montessori approach. Healthcare professionals, including physicians, psychologists, and occupational therapists, can provide valuable insights and expertise in assessing individuals' cognitive abilities, determining appropriate activities, and monitoring their progress.

Collaboration with specialists, such as music therapists, art therapists, or occupational therapists specializing in sensory integration, can further enhance the effectiveness of the Montessori approach. These professionals can offer guidance on incorporating specific therapies or interventions that align with the Montessori principles and complement the overall care plan.

Regular communication and collaboration with healthcare professionals and specialists ensure that individuals' needs are met comprehensively and that care strategies are aligned with the latest research and evidence-based practices. This collaboration enables caregivers to make informed decisions, seek advice, and access additional support when necessary.

Evaluating and adjusting the approach based on individual needs is a continuous and essential process in implementing the Montessori approach. Each individual is unique, with evolving needs and capabilities. Regular assessments and evaluations should be conducted to determine the effectiveness of the approach and make necessary adjustments.

Evaluations can involve monitoring individuals' engagement levels, observing their emotional well-being, and assessing cognitive functioning through standardized assessments or professional observations. Feedback from individuals, family members, and caregivers is also valuable in understanding the impact of the approach and identifying areas for improvement.

Based on evaluation outcomes, caregivers can modify activities, adapt the environment, or seek additional support or expertise as needed. Flexibility and responsiveness are crucial in ensuring that individuals receive the most beneficial and person-centered care.

Implementing the Montessori approach with individuals with dementia and other conditions requires a comprehensive and collaborative effort. Training and education for caregivers provide the necessary knowledge and skills, while adapting physical environments in care facilities and homes create supportive and accessible spaces. Collaboration with healthcare professionals and specialists ensures comprehensive care, and evaluating and adjusting the approach based on individual needs promotes continuous improvement and individualized care. By implementing the Montessori approach with diligence, caregivers can create an environment that promotes independence, engagement, and well-being for individuals with dementia and other conditions.

BENEFITS AND IMPACT OF MONTESSORI APPROACH

A. ENHANCING QUALITY OF LIFE FOR INDIVIDUALS WITH DEMENTIA AND OTHER CONDITIONS

B. IMPROVING COGNITIVE FUNCTIONING AND REDUCING BEHAVIORAL SYMPTOMS

C. PROMOTING EMOTIONAL WELL-BEING AND REDUCING ANXIETY

The Montessori approach has proven to be highly beneficial and impactful when applied to individuals with dementia and other conditions. By emphasizing person-centered care, independence, and tailored activities, the Montessori approach has the potential to significantly enhance the quality of life for individuals with dementia and other conditions.

One of the primary benefits of the Montessori approach for individuals with dementia and other conditions is the enhancement of quality of life. By creating a supportive and engaging environment, individuals are empowered to participate in meaningful activities and maintain a sense of purpose and accomplishment. The Montessori approach recognizes the importance of preserving individuals' dignity and autonomy, which is crucial for promoting overall well-being.

Engaging in the Montessori approach can lead to improved cognitive functioning for individuals with dementia and other conditions. The tailored activities and individualized learning experiences promote cognitive stimulation, memory recall, and problem-solving skills. By providing opportunities for cognitive exercises and brain-stimulating activities, the Montessori approach helps maintain and potentially enhance cognitive abilities, slowing the decline in cognitive functioning.

The Montessori approach has shown promise in reducing behavioral symptoms often associated with dementia and other conditions. By promoting engagement, providing structured routines, and offering meaningful activities, individuals experience a sense of calm and reduced agitation. The focus on independence and autonomy also decreases feelings of frustration and dependence, leading to a more peaceful and harmonious environment.

Promoting emotional well-being and reducing anxiety are additional significant outcomes of the Montessori approach. By incorporating multi-sensory experiences, such as tactile, visual, and auditory stimuli, the approach stimulates the senses and evokes positive emotions. Engaging in social interactions, peer discussions, and intergenerational activities fosters a sense of connection, belonging, and emotional support.

For individuals with conditions such as autism or ADHD, the Montessori approach can alleviate anxiety and provide a structured and predictable environment that supports emotional regulation and self-management. By tailoring activities to match individual preferences and abilities, the approach promotes a sense of confidence, self-esteem, and emotional well-being.

The impact of the Montessori approach extends beyond the individuals themselves. Family members and caregivers also benefit from the approach, as it reduces caregiver burden and enhances the quality of care provided. By implementing the Montessori principles, caregivers experience a shift from a task-focused approach to a person-centered one, resulting in more fulfilling and meaningful interactions.

The Montessori approach has a range of benefits and a significant impact on individuals with dementia and other conditions. By enhancing the quality of life, improving cognitive functioning, reducing behavioral symptoms, and promoting emotional well-being, the approach creates a more supportive and engaging environment for individuals. The person-centered nature of the Montessori approach allows for tailored activities that align with individual strengths, interests, and abilities. By implementing the Montessori principles, caregivers can make a positive difference in the lives of individuals with dementia and other conditions, enhancing their overall well-being and ensuring they maintain a sense of dignity and independence.

CHALLENGES AND CONSIDERATIONS

A. ADAPTING MONTESSORI PRINCIPLES TO DIFFERENT CONDITIONS AND CARE SETTINGS

B. OVERCOMING RESISTANCE AND MISCONCEPTIONS

C. MAINTAINING CONTINUITY AND CONSISTENCY IN IMPLEMENTATION

Adapting Montessori principles to different conditions and care settings can present several challenges and considerations. The successful implementation of the Montessori approach requires overcoming resistance and misconceptions, as well as maintaining continuity and consistency in its application.

One of the primary challenges when adapting Montessori principles to different conditions and care settings is overcoming resistance and misconceptions. The Montessori approach may be perceived as solely applicable to early childhood education, which can lead to skepticism or resistance from caregivers, healthcare professionals, and even individuals themselves. Overcoming these misconceptions requires education and awareness about the adaptability of the Montessori approach across various conditions and care settings.

Caregiver training and professional development programs are crucial in addressing resistance and fostering understanding. By providing comprehensive education on the Montessori approach and its applications in different contexts, caregivers can gain the knowledge and confidence needed to implement it effectively. Additionally, sharing success stories and evidence-based research that demonstrate the positive outcomes of the

Montessori approach in diverse care settings can help overcome resistance and change misconceptions.

Maintaining continuity and consistency in the implementation of the Montessori approach is another significant consideration. As individuals transition between care settings or experience changes in their conditions, it is important to ensure that the principles and strategies of the Montessori approach remain consistent. This requires effective communication, collaboration, and coordination among caregivers, healthcare professionals, and families.

Regular communication channels, such as meetings or digital platforms, can facilitate information sharing and promote a cohesive approach. Caregivers should have access to documentation and guidelines that outline the Montessori principles and how they can be adapted to different conditions and care settings. This ensures that there is a shared understanding of the approach and its implementation across all stakeholders involved in the individual's care.

Another consideration is tailoring the Montessori approach to meet the specific needs and challenges of different conditions and care settings. Each condition has unique characteristics and requires customized approaches to address the individual's specific needs. For example, individuals with dementia may benefit from simplified activities and environmental modifications to support memory recall, while individuals with autism may require structured routines and visual aids to facilitate communication and engagement.

Flexibility and adaptability are essential in implementing the Montessori approach to different conditions and care settings. Caregivers should continuously evaluate and adjust their strategies based on the individual's progress, changing needs, and feedback from the individual, family members, and healthcare professionals. This ongoing assessment ensures that the Montessori approach remains person-centered and responsive to the individual's evolving requirements.

In conclusion, adapting Montessori principles to different conditions and care settings presents challenges and requires careful considerations. Overcoming resistance and misconceptions through education and awareness, as well as maintaining continuity and consistency in implementation through effective communication and coordination, are crucial for success. Tailoring the approach to meet the specific needs of individuals with different conditions and ensuring flexibility and adaptability further enhances its effectiveness. By addressing these challenges and considerations, caregivers can implement the Montessori approach in diverse care settings and positively impact the well-being and quality of life of individuals with various conditions.

CASE STUDIES AND SUCCESS STORIES

A. EXAMPLES OF SUCCESSFUL IMPLEMENTATION IN CARE FACILITIES

B. INDIVIDUAL TESTIMONIALS AND POSITIVE OUTCOMES

Case Study 1: Applying Montessori to Dementia Care

Background: Mrs. Smith is an 80-year-old woman diagnosed with moderate Alzheimer's disease. She resides in a memory care facility where the Montessori approach is implemented.

Application of Montessori Principles:
- Prepared Environment: The facility creates a clear and organized environment for Mrs. Smith. Pathways are free from clutter, and furniture is arranged to promote ease of movement. Labels and visual cues are used to aid navigation.
- Meaningful Activities: Mrs. Smith's preferences, strengths, and abilities are assessed. It is discovered that she has a background in music. Therefore, music therapy sessions are conducted regularly, allowing her to engage in singing, playing musical instruments, and reminiscing about her favorite songs.
- Independence and Autonomy: Mrs. Smith is encouraged to participate in self-care activities, such as dressing and grooming. Adapted materials and tools are provided to support her independence in these tasks.

Outcome: Mrs. Smith shows increased engagement and a sense of purpose. She actively participates in music therapy sessions, demonstrating improved mood and enhanced social interactions. Engaging in self-care activities promotes her independence, leading to improved self-esteem and a sense of accomplishment.

Case Study 2: Applying Montessori to Autism Spectrum Disorder (ASD)

Background: Jake is a 10-year-old boy diagnosed with ASD. He attends a school that implements the Montessori approach, tailored to his specific needs.

Application of Montessori Principles:
• Multi-Sensory Experiences: Jake has sensory sensitivities and prefers tactile stimuli. The environment is adapted to incorporate various tactile materials, such as sand, textured objects, and playdough. These materials are used in activities that promote learning and engagement.
• Individualized Learning: Jake's strengths and interests are assessed. It is discovered that he has a passion for animals. Learning activities are designed around this interest, such as animal-themed puzzles, books, and games.
• Collaboration and Peer Interactions: Group activities are organized to encourage social interactions. Jake participates in cooperative games, group projects, and discussions with his peers,

fostering social connections and communication skills.

Outcome: Jake demonstrates increased engagement and improved social interactions. The incorporation of tactile materials and individualized activities aligned with his interests enhances his learning experience and reduces sensory discomfort. Collaborative activities promote his social skills and provide a sense of belonging within the classroom environment.

Example 1: Montessori Approach for Dementia Care

Background: Mr. Johnson, a 75-year-old man with advanced dementia, resides in a memory care facility that embraces the Montessori approach.

Implementation of the Montessori Approach:
- Prepared Environment: The facility ensures a clear and organized environment for Mr. Johnson. Personal items are placed within reach, and visual cues are used to help him navigate the space independently.
- Meaningful Activities: Mr. Johnson's interests and abilities are assessed, revealing his fondness for gardening. A dedicated garden area is created where he can engage in planting, watering, and tending to plants using adapted tools and clear instructions.

- Social Connections: Group activities and discussions are organized, allowing Mr. Johnson to interact with peers. These activities include reminiscing sessions, where participants share personal stories and engage in meaningful conversations.

-

Positive Outcomes: With the Montessori approach, Mr. Johnson experiences improved mood and engagement. Engaging in gardening activities reduces agitation and enhances his sense of purpose. Social interactions promote a sense of belonging, reduce feelings of isolation, and foster emotional well-being.

Example 2: Montessori Approach for Autism Spectrum Disorder (ASD)

Background: Emma, a 6-year-old girl with ASD, attends a Montessori-inspired school that caters to her specific needs.

Implementation of the Montessori Approach:
- Individualized Learning: Emma's interests and strengths are identified, including her fascination with numbers and patterns. Individualized math activities and materials, such as counting games and pattern blocks, are incorporated into her daily learning routine.

• Multi-Sensory Experiences: Emma has sensory sensitivities, particularly to auditory stimuli. The learning environment is adapted to minimize noise distractions, and headphones are provided when needed. Tactile materials, such as textured fabrics and manipulatives, are used to engage her sense of touch during learning activities.

• Independence and Autonomy: Emma is encouraged to participate in self-care tasks, such as dressing and cleaning up after activities. Visual schedules and step-by-step instructions are provided to support her independence and build her confidence.

Positive Outcomes: Through the Montessori approach, Emma demonstrates increased focus, engagement, and self-regulation. The individualized math activities capitalize on her strengths, fostering a love for learning and improving her numerical skills. The multi-sensory experiences accommodate her sensory sensitivities, reducing anxiety and promoting a more comfortable learning environment. By encouraging her independence, Emma gains a sense of accomplishment and improved self-esteem.

These examples illustrate the successful implementation of the Montessori approach in dementia care and working with individuals with autism spectrum disorder. By tailoring activities to individual interests, promoting independence, and creating supportive environments, positive outcomes such as improved mood, engagement, cognitive functioning, and emotional well-being are achieved. The Montessori approach's person-centered nature allows for customized care that addresses the unique needs and strengths of individuals with dementia and autism spectrum disorder, leading to more fulfilling and meaningful lives.

FUTURE DIRECTIONS AND RESEARCH

A. CONTINUING RESEARCH ON THE EFFICACY OF THE MONTESSORI APPROACH

B. EXPANDING IMPLEMENTATION TO OTHER CONDITIONS AND CARE SETTINGS

C. EXPLORING TECHNOLOGICAL ADVANCEMENTS TO ENHANCE THE APPROACH

The Montessori approach has demonstrated significant benefits when applied to individuals with dementia and other conditions. As the understanding and utilization of the Montessori approach continue to grow, there are ongoing efforts to advance research, expand implementation to other conditions and care settings, and explore technological advancements to enhance its effectiveness.

Continuing Research on the Efficacy of the Montessori Approach:

Researchers and healthcare professionals are continuously conducting studies to assess and validate the efficacy of the Montessori approach for individuals with dementia and other conditions. These studies involve evaluating the impact of the approach on cognitive functioning, emotional well-being, quality of life, and other relevant outcomes.

Research helps identify the specific benefits of the Montessori approach and contributes to evidence-based practices. By examining the mechanisms and underlying principles of the approach, researchers can further refine and tailor interventions to better address the unique needs of individuals with different conditions. Ongoing research also highlights potential areas for improvement and guides the implementation of the Montessori approach in a more targeted and effective manner.

Expanding Implementation to Other Conditions and Care Settings:

While the Montessori approach has been primarily associated with dementia care, there is a growing recognition that its principles can be beneficial for individuals with various other conditions. For instance, individuals with autism spectrum disorder, attention deficit hyperactivity disorder (ADHD), and intellectual disabilities can also benefit from the person-centered and individualized nature of the Montessori approach.

The principles of the Montessori approach can be adapted and implemented in different care settings, such as schools, hospitals, rehabilitation centers, and community-based programs. By expanding the implementation of the Montessori approach to these settings, a broader range of individuals can access its benefits and experience enhanced quality of life.

To ensure successful implementation, training and education programs for caregivers and professionals in these different settings are essential. Such programs can provide the necessary knowledge and skills to apply the Montessori principles effectively, considering the specific needs and characteristics of each condition and care setting.

Exploring Technological Advancements to Enhance the Approach:

Technological advancements offer exciting possibilities for enhancing the implementation of the Montessori approach. Technology can provide innovative tools and platforms to support personalized learning, engagement, and cognitive stimulation for individuals with dementia and other conditions.

For example, digital applications and virtual reality can create immersive and interactive experiences that promote cognitive functioning and engagement. These technologies can be designed to incorporate Montessori-inspired activities and adapt to individual needs, providing a more tailored and dynamic approach.

Additionally, technological advancements can facilitate remote access to Montessori-based interventions, allowing individuals to benefit from the approach even in situations where in-person interactions are limited. Virtual platforms and telehealth services can provide guidance, support, and resources to caregivers and individuals in their homes or remote care settings.

However, it is important to ensure that technological advancements align with the principles of the Montessori approach and do not replace the human connection and interaction that are integral to its success. Technology should be used as a tool to enhance and complement the Montessori approach, rather than replace the personalized and individualized care that it embodies.

The Montessori approach applied to dementia and other conditions continues to evolve and expand. Continuing research contributes to the growing evidence base, allowing for further refinement and customization of interventions. Expanding implementation to other conditions and care settings broadens access to the benefits of the Montessori approach. Exploring technological advancements offers opportunities to enhance the approach through innovative tools and platforms. By embracing these developments, the Montessori approach can continue to positively impact the lives of individuals with dementia and other conditions, promoting cognitive functioning, emotional well-being, and quality of life.

CONCLUSION

The Montessori approach holds significant importance as part of therapy for individuals with dementia and other conditions. Its person-centered care and individualized approach prioritize the unique needs, strengths, and preferences of each individual, fostering a sense of empowerment, engagement, and well-being.

One of the key aspects of the Montessori approach is its person-centered care. It recognizes that every individual is unique and deserves individualized attention and support. This person-centered approach shifts the focus from the condition itself to the individual as a whole person, promoting dignity, respect, and autonomy. By placing the individual's needs, preferences, and abilities at the forefront, the Montessori approach acknowledges their inherent worth and strives to provide personalized care that is meaningful and fulfilling.

Individualization is another fundamental principle of the Montessori approach. It acknowledges that each person has different strengths, interests, and abilities. By tailoring activities, interventions, and the environment to the individual, the Montessori approach recognizes and capitalizes on their unique potential. This individualization fosters a sense of purpose, accomplishment, and satisfaction, which is particularly crucial for individuals with dementia and other conditions who may experience feelings of loss, frustration, or diminished sense of self.

Moreover, the Montessori approach promotes engagement and active participation. It recognizes the importance of meaningful activities and experiences that align with the individual's interests and abilities. By providing purposeful and engaging tasks, the Montessori approach stimulates cognitive functioning, maintains or enhances skills, and promotes a sense of accomplishment. This engagement is critical for individuals with dementia and other conditions, as it supports cognitive stimulation, social interaction, emotional well-being, and overall quality of life.

Additionally, the Montessori approach emphasizes the empowerment and independence of individuals. It encourages individuals to actively participate in their care, decision-making, and daily activities to the best of their abilities. By providing opportunities for choice, autonomy, and self-direction, the Montessori approach promotes a sense of control and self-confidence, even in the face of cognitive decline or other challenges. This empowerment fosters a positive self-image and helps individuals maintain a sense of identity and agency.

The Montessori approach also recognizes the importance of creating a supportive and enabling environment. It focuses on adapting physical spaces, materials, and activities to meet the specific needs of individuals. By modifying the environment to support independence, accessibility, and safety, the Montessori approach ensures that individuals can engage in activities with minimal barriers. This environment fosters a sense of security, familiarity, and freedom, allowing individuals to navigate and participate actively in their surroundings.

In conclusion, the Montessori approach is of utmost importance as part of therapy for individuals with dementia and other conditions. By recognizing the inherent worth of each individual and tailoring interventions to their specific needs, the Montessori approach provides a foundation for meaningful and fulfilling therapy.